Fatma Khalsi

Bronchopulmonary malformations in children

Fatma Khalsi

Bronchopulmonary malformations in children

ScienciaScripts

Imprint

Any brand names and product names mentioned in this book are subject to trademark, brand or patent protection and are trademarks or registered trademarks of their respective holders. The use of brand names, product names, common names, trade names, product descriptions etc. even without a particular marking in this work is in no way to be construed to mean that such names may be regarded as unrestricted in respect of trademark and brand protection legislation and could thus be used by anyone.

Cover image: www.ingimage.com

This book is a translation from the original published under ISBN 978-620-6-71384-5.

Publisher:
Sciencia Scripts
is a trademark of
Dodo Books Indian Ocean Ltd. and OmniScriptum S.R.L publishing group

120 High Road, East Finchley, London, N2 9ED, United Kingdom
Str. Armeneasca 28/1, office 1, Chisinau MD-2012, Republic of Moldova, Europe
Printed at: see last page
ISBN: 978-620-7-68800-5

CONTENTS

Introduction

Congenital pulmonary malformations are rare (1) and constitute a very varied group encompassing anomalies linked to the development of the tracheobronchial tree.

They are secondary to an abnormality in embryonic lung development and are formed between 6 and 17 weeks of amenorrhoea.

They have the same embryological origin; however, their clinical presentation, histology and management differ from one malformation to another.

These malformations are discovered in childhood during an infectious episode or respiratory distress.

Their overall frequency is difficult to establish, as they may remain asymptomatic until adolescence.(1).

In Tunisia, few studies have focused on MBPs.

According to the literature, the most common are adenomatoid cystic malformations

(MAKP), pulmonary hypoplasia, bronchogenic cysts (KB) and giant lobar emphysema (GLE)(1)

Early diagnosis is desirable thanks to morphological ultrasound, which makes neonatal treatment possible.

Imaging (chest X-ray, CT scan, thoracic ultrasound, MRI, etc.) is essential to confirm the diagnosis.

Multidisciplinary management is required to obtain an accurate diagnosis and

adopt the best treatment strategy, based essentially on surgery.

I.   Reminder of the development of the respiratory tree

I.1 Stages and physiology of tracheobronchopulmonary development :

I.1.1 Stages of lung development :

Around day 24 to 26, the primitive digestive tract (primitive intestine) duplicates and produces a longitudinal diverticulum on its anterior surface: the respiratory diverticulum.

 The oesophageal-tracheal septum then forms. The trachea, thus separated from the oesophagus, divides from 5 SA: 23 generations of dichotomous divisions. These buds, accompanied by a mesodermal component, develop in the coelomic cavity (future pleural cavities). The pulmonary arteries, originating from the sixth aortic arch, are located in the mesenchyme surrounding the epithelial outline; they follow the development of the air ducts.

Lung development takes place in five distinct morphological and functional stages.

Different stages of lung development

Stade	Période	Évènements
Embryonnaire	0-7 semaines	Émergence du bourgeon pulmonaire Premières ramifications bronchiques Acquisition de l'asymétrie droite-gauche Naissance des gros vaisseaux (artère et veine pulmonaires)
Pseudoglandulaire	8-16 semaines	Formation de l'arbre bronchique par segmentations successives Développement parallèle de l'arbre vasculaire
Canaliculaire	16-27 semaines	Formation des acini, dernières divisions terminales Différenciation des épithéliums proximal et distal Différenciation des pneumocytes I et II Amincissement du parenchyme Formation d'une barrière « primitive » d'échanges
Sacculaire	28-25 semaines	Formation des saccules, expansion des espaces aériens Accumulation des inclusions lamellaires Capillaires au contact de la membrane basale
Alvéolaire	Terme à 3 ans	Formation des alvéoles par septalisation secondaire Fusion des capillaires, passage à un seul système capillaire Amincissement ultime de la barrière d'échange

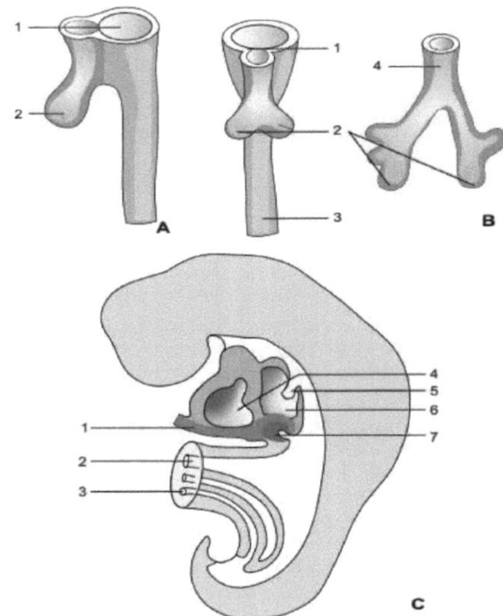

A. **Primary intestine:**
(Around the 6th week)
1. foregut
2. Respiratory diverticulum.

B. **Oesotracheal septum and first bronchial divisions :**
1. Oesotracheal septum
2. Bronchial buds
3. Oesophagus
4. Trachea.

C. **Schematic view of the thoracic cavity** :
(Around the 5th week)
1. Septum transversum
2. Yolk duct
3. Allantoid
4. Pericardial cavity
5. Tracheal bud
6. Pleural cavity
7. Liver bud

Development of lung buds(3)

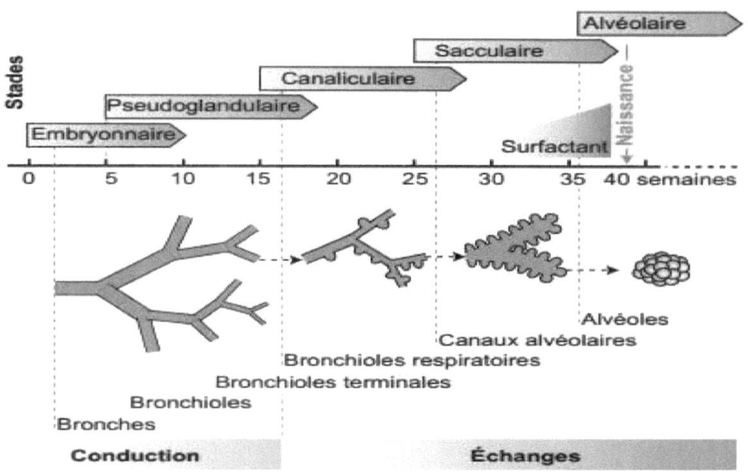

I.1.2 Specific features of postnatal growth

a. Alveolus growth

After the age of 2 to 4, the alveoli increase in size until the thorax stops growing. The volume of the lung increases 20-fold between birth and adulthood.

b. Bronchial growth

The bronchial tubes change postnatally as the body grows, with an increase in their calibre and length. Bronchial cartilage is thought to develop for up to 2 years.

c. Installation of collateral ventilation

Kohn's pores appear after birth, Lambert's ducts around the age of 8.

d. Growth of the pulmonary circulation

The structure of the pulmonary artery walls changes: their thickness is halved between birth and the age of 6 months to 2 years, and muscularisation progresses towards the distal airways over time.

I.1.3 Physiological factors in lung development

a. Fetal lung fluid

Experimental work has demonstrated the existence of a clean pulmonary fluid secreted by the pulmonary epithelium, contained in the bronchial lumen and evacuated via the trachea, either by discharge into the amniotic fluid or by swallowing.

This secretion is thought to be linked to active transfers of chlorine ions across the pulmonary epithelium and is influenced by endocrine factors, hypoxia and foetal respiratory movements.

b. Fetal respiratory movements :

From the first trimester onwards, these thoracic movements lead to displacements of pulmonary fluid in the trachea (inducing pressure variations in the air spaces), and are essentially due to the action of the diaphragm and other respiratory muscles. Their role in the development of the foetal lung is certain. They are of great importance, since sectioning the phrenic nerves in animals leads to pulmonary hypoplasia.(4)

c. Lung expansion volume :

In order to develop, the lungs need sufficient intrathoracic (and indirectly intrauterine) space. The pulmonary hypoplasia observed in severe hydrops proves this. In addition, any fetal thoracic or abdominal compression interferes with diaphragmatic clearance, and therefore fetal respiratory movements, which exacerbates the developmental anomaly of the fetal lung.

d. Lung pressures :

The balance between pressures and volumes within the airspaces is essential for the proper development of the lungs. An increase in intraluminal pressure leads to a reduction in the secretion of intrapulmonary fluid.

e. Lung biochemical maturation :

This is the acquisition by the epithelial cells of the ability to secrete pulmonary surfactant. Surfactant regulates alveolar homeostasis and prevents the alveoli from collapsing.(5).

I.2 Mechanisms regulating tracheobronchopulmonary development :

The physical environment of the lung plays a major role at every stage of its development.

I.2.1 Genetic control :

Several developmental genes are involved throughout lung morphogenesis. For example, NKX2.1, HNF-3b and GATA play an important role in the individualisation of the tracheal outline. Lefty-1 is important for the acquisition of lung asymmetry. Other genes are also important: bmp4 and FGF-10 in the bronchial branches, Shh in the tracheo-oesophageal separation, factors of the transforming growth factor [TGF] family: invalidation of the TGF-b3 gene is associated with arrest of lung development at the pseudo-glandular stage; platelet derived growth factor, invalidation of which is responsible for late arrest of development at the alveolisation stage.

I.2.2 The extracellular matrix :

Many components of the extracellular matrix (collagen, laminins, proteoglycans, fibronectins) play an essential role in lung morphogenesis. These molecules recognise membrane receptors called integrins. Invalidation of the gene encoding one of the integrin 3 subunits abolishes binding to laminin 5 and disrupts the branching process.

I.2.3 Endothelial cells :

Recent advances in vascular biology have highlighted the importance of the endothelial cell in the development and vasomotor regulation of the pulmonary circulation. Regulation of pulmonary vasomotor tone in the perinatal period results from a balance between vasodilator and vasoconstrictor mediators released by the endothelial cell. Among these substances, NO and endothelin-1 (ET-1) play a major role. Invalidation of the NOS-3 gene in mice induces pulmonary arterial hypertension and increased pulmonary vasoconstriction in response to hypoxia. Its role in the physiological regulation of pulmonary vasomotor tone in the foetus is not well established.

I.2.4 Mesenchyme-epithelium interaction :

From the embryonic period, mesenchyme plays a fundamental inductive role in the processes of branching and epithelial differentiation. Grafting of distal mesenchyme onto tracheal epithelium induces branching and the expression of alveolar markers. Grafting of tracheal mesenchyme onto distal epithelium inhibits branching and induces expression of a mucociliary epithelium.

I.3 Hormonal regulation of lung maturation :

I.3.1 Glucocorticoids :

The physiological acceleration of lung maturation in the last weeks of the saccular period is associated with an increase in cortisol production by the adrenal cortex. Glucocorticoids contribute to normal surfactant maturation.

I.3.2 Thyroid hormones :

The effect of thyroid hormones on lung maturation is well established experimentally. The lungs of rabbit foetuses treated with thyroxine have better aeration, a greater number of lamellar inclusions and accelerated morphological maturation. Thyroid hormones increase surfactant phospholipid levels and have a significant effect on lung growth, particularly on septal formation.

I.3.3 Beta-adrenergic agonists :

Cyclic adenosine monophosphorus (AMP), phosphodiesterase inhibitors and beta-adrenergic agonists increase the synthesis and secretion of phosphatidylcholine. Cyclic AMP is a direct activator of transcription of the surfactant SP-A protein gene.

I.4 Pathophysiological hypotheses :

I.4.1 Bronchovascular anomaly :

The hypothesis of a single bronchovascular anomaly at the origin of bronchopulmonary malformations as proposed by Clements and Warner seems attractive (6). The cause would be a lesion at the end of the bronchial tree, the aetiology of which is variable, in the form of localised trauma, ischaemia or infection. Moreover, it is not only the nature of the attack, but above all the date of onset and severity that will determine t h e   morphological appearance of the lesion. It is therefore often a malformative spectrum as described by Achiron et al. (7)ranging from a normal lung vascularised by normal or non-normal vessels to an abnormal lung, i.e. a dysplastic lung vascularised by normal or non-normal vessels.

I.4.2 Cell proliferation abnormality(8)

Cass et al proposed the hypothesis of a disturbance in cell proliferation; they showed that, in MAKP, the index of cell proliferation was twice as high as in normal lung (foetal or neonatal), while the index of apoptosis was five times lower, the more extensive the lesion. These abnormalities in the regulation of cell proliferation are under the control of multiple growth factors, the mechanisms of which have yet to be fully elucidated.

I.4.3 Obstructive hypothesis :

The histological study of pulmonary malformations led Langston to propose the hypothesis of an obstructive sequence at the origin of these malformations (9). This hypothesis is based on several observations. On the one hand, the coexistence of several pulmonary malformations in the same patient is regularly described. Secondly, the presence of small cysts, identical to those seen in MAKP, is also found in bronchial atresia and extra-lobar sequestration. These observations therefore suggest a common mechanism at the origin of malformative processes. Cystic dilatations could be secondary to an organic (bronchial stenosis) or functional (abnormal peristalsis) obstacle in the airways(9). Differences in appearance

would be related to the location, degree and timing of airway obstruction (10).

I.4.4 Lung development abnormalities

The localised nature of the pulmonary malformations, the normality of the upstream and downstream lung and the persistent expression within these malformations of markers of early pulmonary development such as thyroid transcription factor-1 (TTF-1) or Hox b5 suggest the hypothesis of a localised and transient anomaly of pulmonary development, occurring during the pseudo-glandular (6 to 16 SA) or canalicular (17 to 26 SA) stages(11,12).

Lung development is the result of permanent reciprocal interactions between the epithelial and mesenchymal components of the lung bud. These interactions are mediated by factors that are diffusible between these two compartments. MAKP could result from abnormal interactions between the epithelium and mesenchyme(13). It is in fact possible in vitro and in vivo to induce cystic dilatations of the airways by overexpressing factors involved in lung development such as fibroblast growth factor 10 (FGF-10), FGF-7 and transforming growth factor (TGF)-1(14)

I.4.5 Obstruction and developmental abnormality

The obstructive and developmental hypotheses are not contradictory. The experiment by Unbekandt et al summarises them, showing that FGF-10 expression can be induced by a mechanical stimulus(15). Tracheal occlusion of fetal mouse lung in culture causes an increase in pressure in the airways and induces a diffuse increase in FGF-10 expression. It is therefore likely that a local increase in airway pressure is capable of inducing a local increase in FGF-10 expression. This would induce localised dilation of the air tree until the level of FGF-10 expression returns to its basal level thanks to retrocontrol mechanisms, allowing normal budding to continue.

Others suggest a hypothesis involving fibroblast growth factor (FGF)10 at the origin of congenital cystic malformations of the lung. An initial anomaly in FGF-10 acts on foetal bronchial tone and creates functional bronchial obstruction, generating a vicious malformative circle. However, the mode of entry into this circle remains unknown(16).

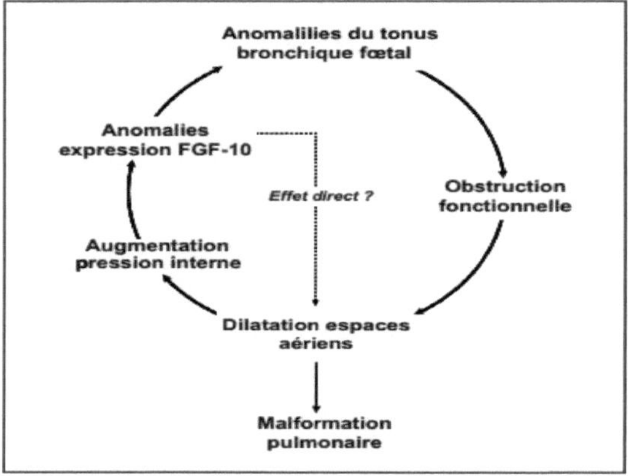

Pathogenic hypothesis according to HADCHOUEL(16)

II.   Epidemiology

II.1 Frequency

Congenital bronchopulmonary malformations (BPM) are rare, and their overall frequency is difficult to establish because they may remain asymptomatic and unrecognised.(1). In the literature, an annual incidence of 30-42 cases per 100,000 population has been reported (16,17).

According to the literature, the most common BPMs are cystic adenomatoid malformations (CAAM), giant lobar emphysema (GLE), pulmonary sequestration (PS) and bronchogenic cysts (BK).(1).

II.2 Gender

The gender distribution varied from one series to another. No predominance of one gender over the other was reported.

III. Clinic

III.1 Neonatal period

In a minority of cases, CPB can lead to severe respiratory complications at birth, requiring mechanical ventilation and immediate surgical intervention. Prenatal assessment of the risk of neonatal respiratory distress is essential to help decide where mothers should be delivered. The studies available on this subject are often limited by an imprecise definition of neonatal respiratory symptoms, their retrospective and monocentric nature, or the small number of patients. The most accurate data comes from the French database developed by the reference centre for rare respiratory diseases in children (RespiRare®). This study shows that 25% of children with a prenatal diagnosis of CPB had respiratory symptoms at birth, 13% required oxygen administration, and 11% required respiratory assistance. The main predictors of neonatal respiratory distress were signs of prenatal compression, and above all a malformational volume to head circumference ratio (CVR) greater than 0.84. However, there are limitations to this study, which prevent these markers from being applied routinely: non-exhaustive postnatal inclusion of children, retrospective recording of prenatal data. The prospective MALFPULM study, currently underway, will help to avoid recruitment bias, and to obtain complete and reproducible prenatal parameters.

The MALFPULM study is the first comprehensive prospective study of this disease. It will be the largest cohort ever published of children with CPM. This study is possible thanks to the motivation of all those involved in monitoring these malformations: obstetricians in CPDPNs, paediatric surgeons and paediatric respirologists. It provides a complete description of the natural history of these malformations, from their discovery in the womb, which limits the biases induced by purely postnatal recruitment.

Its results will have a direct impact on public health, by validating a prognostic model that will provide better guidance for the care of women whose foetus is affected by SCD, and in particular by helping to decide where these mothers should give birth.

It is also a unique opportunity to prospectively collect malformation tissue from surgical resections, and to assess for the first time, in a large, perfectly phenotyped cohort, the true frequency of oncogenic K-ras mutations in the epithelial cells lining malformation cysts.

In just over a year, 150 children have already been included. This figure only confirms the motivation of the teams and the interest of this study, while underlining once again the limitations of the Respirare cohort, which collected only 85 children over 3 years.

III.2 Complications after birth

For the majority of children born with CPB, no respiratory complications are observed at birth, or even during the first few years of life. There is debate about the need for elective surgery in these asymptomatic children. In a British cohort, infection is rare in the first five years. The French Respirare data confirms the exceptional nature of infection in the first two years, but highlights a high risk of wheezing, which persists after surgery. The hypothesis of bronchial hyperresponsiveness associated with the malformation has been put forward (Delestrain et al, submitted). Systematic removal of these malformations would be mainly justified by the prevention of their potential malignant transformation. More than 20 cases associating MAKP and bronchioloalveolar carcinoma (BAC) have been reported over the last 20 years, as young as 8 years of age. Intracystic islands of mucus cells, with mutations in codon 12 of the KRAS gene, have been described in type 1 MAKP, making these lesions potential precursors of BAC. However, it is far from certain that any type 1 MAKP is a pre-cancerous lesion. Mucinous islands are inconstant, identified in 26% to 50% of type 1 MPAK, and the presence of KRAS mutations has not been confirmed in another series of 34 MPC.

IV. Adenomatoid cystic pulmonary malformations (ACPM) or congenital malformations of the pulmonary airways

CPAMs are characterised by abnormal lung tissue (a hamartomatous mass of disorganised lung tissue evolving into a more or less cystic mass) linked to a localised maturation arrest of the bronchial tree. In 2002, Stocker proposed the use of the term Congenital Pulmonary Airway Malformations (CPAM) and described 5 types depending on the site of airway involvement: type 0 (tracheobronchial, incompatible with life), type 1 (bronchi or bronchioles), type 2 (bronchioles), type 3 (bronchioles or alveolar ducts), type 4 (acinar, the most distal). The disease most often affects a single lobe, but bi-lobar and even bilateral forms also exist. All lobes may be affected, but the lesion is more frequently found in the lower lobes. Sequestration is a frequent association, reported in around 25% of cases (hybrid forms). Some authors have reported associated urinary, digestive and cardiac malformations, which are more frequent in type 2. Recent literature shows that MAKP is rarely associated with extra-thoracic malformations.

IV.1 Clinical :

In the neonatal period, the most frequent clinical picture is the presence of respiratory signs ranging from polypnoea to respiratory distress, but most patients are asymptomatic during this period. Cases of neonatal pneumothorax have been reported. After the neonatal period, the most frequent mode of revelation is repeated pulmonary infections that can lead to pulmonary abscesses.

IV.2 Imaging :

Currently, the diagnosis of MAKP is based on antenatal imaging, and postnatal diagnoses have become exceptional. Antenatal imaging suggests the diagnosis when there are multiple intrapulmonary cystic images with no abnormality of the diaphragmatic dome, or when there is a hyperechoic lesion on ultrasound and a T2 hypersignal lesion on MRI, with no visible systemic vascularisation within the lesion. Antenatal assessment is used to determine the extent of the lesion and to assess the prognosis. Large lesions cause mediastinal compression, which may be complicated by hydramnios or hydrops. The appearance of hydrops is a poor prognostic factor with a high risk of death. In the absence of hydrops, but when the mediastinal deviation is significant and persists at the end of pregnancy, the risk of neonatal respiratory distress is high, requiring treatment at birth in a specialised environment. The risk of pulmonary hypoplasia in MAKP is rare in the absence of associated complications or malformations, despite the large lesions observed during the second trimester of pregnancy. This could be explained by the natural evolution of MAKP, which frequently decreases in size during the third trimester. Some cases of antenatal regression have been described. In our experience, the postnatal X-ray is normal, but the CT scan often reveals small lesions.

Postnatally, there are several radiological aspects:

- Homogeneous pulmonary condensation with no detectable cystic image. This appearance is more frequently seen in type 3 or in the immediate neonatal period before the cysts aerate.

- Multiple cystic images of variable size, with thin walls.

- Association of cystic images and areas of pulmonary condensation. This is the most common radiological appearance.

- Single cystic image.

Whatever the radiological appearance, there may be a mediastinal shift on the side opposite the lesion. In the case of infectious complications, water-air levels appear within the cystic cavities and the cyst wall becomes thick. Chest X-rays underestimate the lesions, and CT scans are the gold standard. CT confirms the diagnosis by showing the presence of thin-walled cysts. It provides details of the extent of the lesions. It looks for complications: intra-cystic water-aerated levels, thick cyst walls, areas of consolidation, ventilatory problems. Finally, it will look for sequestration, which is often associated.

In the absence of a known history of malformation, complicated forms of MAKP are difficult to differentiate in the acute period from infectious pneumonia. In the neonatal period, the presence of intra-thoracic cystic lesions should rule out the diagnosis of diaphragmatic hernia. Ultrasound in this context is essential to check the position of the abdominal viscera and look for a diaphragmatic defect. Long-term evolution is always marked by complications. Infectious complications are the most frequent. Respiratory distress due to cyst enlargement is less common. Finally, there are cases of

exceptional cases of degeneration have been described. MAKP is treated surgically. Total excision is essential to avoid recurrence, but it must be sparing, which requires an accurate and early assessment of extension, as the increase in cyst volume may overestimate the volume of the lesion. Surgery is performed urgently if respiratory distress is threatening. In the absence of symptoms, most teams recommend surgery at around 5 to 6 months of age, in order to limit the anaesthetic risk, restrict the resection to pathological areas before any infectious complications and improve the prognosis for lung function, as alveolar growth at this age is still significant, allowing compensation for the areas operated on.

V.   Lung sequestration

Sequestrations are characterised by an abnormal pulmonary territory which has lost its normal connections with the bronchial tree and whose arterial vascularisation is of the systemic type. The artery vascularising the malformation arises from the aorta or one of its branches. Two types of sequestration are classically described: intra-lobar sequestration (ILS) and extra-lobar sequestration (ELS). In SIL, the malformation is an integral part of the healthy lung parenchyma, with venous return taking place within the pulmonary system. In SEL, the malformation is surrounded by a clean pleura, and venous drainage is via the vena cava or azygos. SIL is the most common type. Exceptionally, atypical sequestrations are described, associating complex anomalies; in particular, the sequestrated territory may communicate with the oesophagus via a true oesophageal bronchus. Congenital sequestration occurs almost exclusively in the lower lobes. SEL may be subdiaphragmatic. Bilateral forms exist. An important point that we have already emphasised is the frequent association of sequestrations with MAKP (CPAM), as demonstrated by anatomopathological studies of surgical specimens.

V.1 Clinical :

At birth, sequestrations are usually asymptomatic, except in cases of associated malformations, particularly cardiac. Cases of heart failure or pulmonary arterial hypertension have been reported in cases of significant vascular shunting. In infants and children, SEL is most often discovered by chance, whereas SIL is revealed by persistent pneumopathy or recurrent pneumopathy. Cases of haemoptysis have been reported in older children and adults.

V.2 Imaging :

The diagnosis is very often made antenatally in the presence of a hyperechoic lesion on ultrasound with visualisation of an abnormal systemic arterial pedicle on ultrasound or MRI.

Post-natal chest X-rays show :

- in the case of SEL, a homogeneous opacity posing the problem of a mass in the absence of a known malformation,

- in the case of SIL, pulmonary condensation or a heterogeneous opacity with ill-defined contours suggestive of a focus of pneumopathy which does not clear up despite well-administered medical treatment.

When the diagnosis has been made antenatally, the chest X-ray may be normal at birth, but this should not rule out the diagnosis if a lesion existed in utero.

On CT scan, sequestrations classically appear as a mass in the case of SEL or an area of pulmonary condensation with aerated zones in the case of SIL. Some LTS may be aerated if they communicate with the oesophagus. Some SILs show a subnormal appearance of the lung parenchyma or a hyperenlightened appearance. The presence of cystic images should suggest a hybrid form.

In all cases, diagnosis is based on identification of the abnormal systemic vascular pedicle.

Ultrasound and Doppler can easily be used to visualise this abnormal vessel when it arises from the abdominal aorta or one of its branches. When the vessel arises from the thoracic aorta, a CT scan with contrast medium injection is used to visualise the arterial pedicle and to study venous return. A CT scan should explore the entire thorax and the upper part of the abdominal cavity, up to the level of the celiac trunk, which may give rise to the abnormal arterial pedicle. MRI visualises the vascular pedicle, but CT should be preferred to MRI because CT can be used to search for MAKP or other associated malformations.

The therapeutic management of pulmonary sequestrations is not unequivocal in the literature, as cases of complete regression have been reported. However, these malformations may become superinfected and, above all, they may be associated with a MAKP in pathological anatomy, which, according to some authors, justifies their removal. The principle is to perform a sectional ligation of the abnormal systemic vessel, combined with excision of the parenchymal territory. Some authors suggest embolisation of the systemic artery.

VI. Bronchogenic cysts

Bronchogenic cysts are congenital cystic masses of the mediastinum or, more rarely, intra-pulmonary cystic masses. They arise from a defect in the organisation of the tracheobronchial tract and therefore develop in contact with the trachea, bronchi or intestine (the tracheobronchial axis developing from the primitive intestine). The contents of the cysts may be fluid or mucoid.

In pathological anatomy, the cyst is lined with respiratory-type epithelium, making it possible to differentiate it from an oesophageal cystic duplication. However, it is sometimes difficult to differentiate these two entities, even on histology.

VI.1 Clinical :

Bronchogenic cysts may be asymptomatic or revealed by a variety of respiratory signs ranging from coughing to respiratory distress. Clinical signs depend on the location of the cyst, its size and whether or not it communicates with the bronchial tree.

VI.2 Imaging :

The diagnosis is currently made in utero, but some cysts are discovered postnatally. The most common appearance is that of a single, rounded mass with clean margins that appears as a round opacity on a chest X-ray. Ultrasound, when the cyst is accessible, can confirm the fluid nature of the lesion. Computed tomography shows a hypodense lesion, which may be denser if the cyst contents are mucoid. Injection of contrast does not show enhancement. On MRI, bronchogenic cysts show a T2 hypersignal and a variable signal on T1-weighted sequences. The existence of a communication with the bronchial tree, either congenital or, more often, acquired after superinfection, leads to the appearance of a hydroaeric level which, in the absence of a clinical context, leads to the diagnosis of an abscess. More rarely, the appearance is that of an aerial cyst which may become compressive through a "check valve" mechanism. The wall of a cyst may become calcified during inflammatory complications.

It is important to note that bronchogenic cysts are not associated with vertebral malformations, which contrasts with neuro-enteric cysts.

VI.3 Topographical shapes

Right paratracheal cysts are the most common. They are very often asymptomatic, discovered by chance. These cysts may extend posteriorly or even intertracheo-oesophageally.

Because of their location and size, subcarinal or hilar cysts can cause bronchial compression, leading to obstructive emphysema or, more rarely, atelectasis. Small subcarinal cysts are difficult to diagnose, and the chest X-ray should show an opening in the carina with horizontalization of the bronchial tubes. Retrocardial cysts of the lower mediastinum are often asymptomatic. Their relationship and close connections with the oesophagus explain the possibility of oesophageal symptoms. Intraparenchymal bronchogenic cysts can be found in any lobe and present as solitary pulmonary nodules. In the absence of complications, they are asymptomatic.

Given the risk of infection, surgical treatment is always considered, and the pre-operative work-up should include a CT scan rather than an MRI scan to check for pulmonary complications and associated malformations.

VII.   Giant lobar emphysema (GLE)

This pulmonary malformation is characterised by distension of a lobe, several lobes or a pulmonary segment. Classically, ELG preferentially affects the left upper lobe, the middle lobe and the right upper lobe. Localisation in the lower lobes is more rarely described.

Anatomopathologically, two forms have been described: type I, the most common, and type II. In all cases, there is no destruction of the lung parenchyma and the term emphysema is misleading. In type I, the distended lung has normal pulmonary architecture, the radial alveolar count is normal for the age, but the size of the alveoli and alveolar collars is 3 to 10 times greater than normal. In some areas, there may be a rupture of the inter-alveolar partitions. In type II, also known as poly-alveolar lung, the distension is more modest, the size but above all the number of alveoli is increased, with a radial alveolar count greater than +2DS for age.

In almost half of cases, no aetiology is found. In the other cases, we need to look for congenital bronchial stenosis or bronchial cartilage abnormalities.

VII.1 Clinical :

It is common to read that the diagnosis is made in the neonatal period or in the first few months of life in the presence of respiratory signs ranging from polypnoea to respiratory distress. Antenatal diagnosis, the development of imaging techniques and the monitoring of the evolution of ELG have modified these clinical data, and recent literature shows that symptoms may be delayed or that ELG may have no clinical translation.

VII.2 Imaging :

The diagnosis can be made antenatally in the presence of a hyperechoic lesion on ultrasound and a T2 hypersignal lesion on MRI. If normal pulmonary arterial vessels are found within the lesion, the diagnosis of bronchial obstruction can be made in utero. The risk of neonatal respiratory distress is all the greater if the lesion is large and responsible for mediastinal deviation on scans performed at the end of pregnancy.

In the hours following birth, ELG appears on standard radiography as a lobar opacity. The opacity is due to the persistence of unabsorbed pulmonary fluid within the lesion. Computed tomography shows ground-glass images associated with thickening of the interlobular septa, linked to resorption of alveolar fluid by lymphatic channels. Ultrasound showed an echogenic lung, with harmonious pulmonary-type vascularisation on Doppler.

The characteristic post-natal appearance is that of obstructive emphysema. A frontal X-ray of the lung shows a hyperenlightened, distended lobe with opposite-sided mediastinal collapse. When the distension is severe, the X-ray shows a large, hyper-clear lung with contralateral mediastinal collapse and atelectasis of the adjacent lobes. The expiratory film confirms the existence of trapping in the affected lobe(s).

Computed tomography confirms the diagnosis, showing a distended, hyper-clear lobe with vascular rarefaction. Exhalation slices and multiplanar reconstructions can be used to look for bronchial stenosis or bronchomalacia, which are easier to diagnose endoscopically. Computed tomography plays a fundamental role in ruling out obstructive emphysema secondary to extrinsic compression of the bronchus by a mediastinal mass, an abnormal vessel or, more exceptionally, secondary to an endoluminal bronchial lesion. In infants, the main cause of obstructive emphysema is a bronchial foreign body. In general, the clinical context is suggestive and the diagnosis is made based on the notion of a penetration syndrome with sudden onset of dyspnoea.

When the diagnosis was made antenatally, the chest X-ray may be normal and the CT scan showed only a small, localised, hyperclar lesion. In our experience, most of the hyperechoic lesions seen antenatally and regressing postnatally correspond to segmental localised emphysema or bronchial atresia, the exact nature of which is difficult to ascertain because these children do not undergo surgery.

If the child is symptomatic, surgical treatment with lobectomy is necessary. If the child is asymptomatic, simple monitoring is considered, as some lobar emphysema regresses. Lung scintigraphy can help with therapeutic management by studying the functional value of the affected lobe.

VIII. Bronchial atresia

This pulmonary malformation is characterised by the complete interruption of a

bronchus. Downstream of the atresia, the pulmonary structures are normal and are

ventilated postnatally by collateral airways: Kohn's pores and Lambert's ducts.

Bronchial secretions gradually accumulate in the post-atresic cul-de-sac, which

gradually fills with fluid and produces a bronchocele. All bronchi may be affected.

In pathological anatomy, it is sometimes difficult to confirm the diagnosis of

bronchial atresia if longitudinal sections of the pathological bronchus are not

taken.

VIII.1 Clinical :

In newborns, this malformation is asymptomatic. The absence of symptoms may

persist into adulthood, and it is most often discovered incidentally in children.

VIII.2 Imaging

The diagnosis can be made antenatally. The appearance is similar to that seen in

giant lobar emphysema. The parenchymal anomaly is the consequence of a

bronchial obstruction, incomplete in giant lobar emphysema, complete in

bronchial atresia. Postnatally, the characteristic imaging appearance is the

association of obstructive emphysema localised to the pathological territory and

a rounded parahilar opacity corresponding to the bronchocele. In infants, the image of a bronchocele may be absent or small and not visible on the chest X-ray. In the hours following birth, the lesion may appear as a parenchymal opacity in the pathological territory due to the delayed resorption of alveolar fluid in this territory, or the X-ray may be normal if the lesion is very localised.

Computed tomography is the most effective examination for showing the bronchocele, visible as a rounded or fusiform opacity, within which there may be air or a hydro-aerosic level. The lung parenchyma in contact with the bronchocele is hyper-clear with vascular rarefaction and expiratory sections show the existence of expiratory trapping. Bronchial endoscopy confirms the diagnosis if the atresia is in a lobar or segmental bronchus. Long-term evolution is marked by the appearance of respiratory signs and episodes of superinfection. The fact that this malformation is usually asymptomatic in children raises the problem of treatment. Some authors recommend simple surveillance, while others recommend surgical removal to avoid long-term complications.

IX. Tracheal agenesis and atresia

It is part of the CHAOS syndrome (Congenital High Airway Obstruction Syndrome). It is a rare malformation, often fatal. In agenesis, the trachea is completely absent, whereas in atresia, the trachea is partially in place but not permeable. In all cases, there is an interruption between the trachea and the bronchi, responsible during foetal life for retention of pulmonary fluid downstream of the obstacle. The diagnosis must be made in utero on the basis of imaging data. Ultrasound shows two large hyperechoic lungs within which there may be cystic images associated with dilated bronchi filled with pulmonary fluid. Distension of the lungs causes eversion of the diaphragm and mediastinal compression, and ascites is often associated. Cardiac compression and impaired venous return are responsible for anasarca. MRI confirms the ultrasound findings. The lungs are large, with a homogeneous T2 hypersignal, and the dilated bronchi are visible as fluid images. MRI confirms the diagnosis by showing an interruption of the trachea, which is normally always visualised along its entire length, with a liquid T2 hypersignal. Associated cardiovascular, gastrointestinal and genitourinary malformations are common. The severity of this malformation usually leads to termination of pregnancy. In the Anglo-Saxon literature, some authors suggest in utero surgical procedures or EXIT procedures for delivery.

X. Lung agenesis and aplasia

Lung agenesis or aplasia is characterised by the total absence of a lung, due to the arrested development of a bronchial bud. In the case of pulmonary aplasia, a rudimentary stem bronchus remains, with no lung tissue or vessels. Lung agenesis or aplasia may be isolated or may form part of a poly-malformative syndrome associating multiple lesions: bone, digestive, cardiac, urinary or of the contralateral lung. In isolated forms, the prognosis for right-sided lung agenesis is worse than that for left-sided lung agenesis, because in right-sided agenesis there is greater distortion of the large vessels of the mediastinum. Diagnosis is currently made antenatally. Antenatal imaging must carefully study the contralateral lung. Apart from associated lesions, hypoplasia of the single lung is a poor prognostic factor and it is therefore necessary to calculate lung volume in the ante-natal period. Post-natal forms are often discovered by chance. X-rays show a dark, retractile hemithorax with a large contralateral lung leading to mediastinal deviation. Postnatally, the only differential diagnosis is pulmonary atelectasis, which should be investigated by ultrasound. A CT scan is used to differentiate between agenesis and aplasia and to look for associated pulmonary malformations.

XI.   Lobar agenesis, lobar aplasia, pulmonary hypoplasia

These malformations are all characterised by a small lung. They are divided into two groups:

The group of agenesis, lobar aplasia and the group of pulmonary hypoplasia. We recall two embryological notions, already described in. Firstly, the development of the pulmonary vessels is induced by the development of the tracheobronchial bud. Consequently, the complete absence of development of a lobar bronchial bud responsible for lobar agenesis is always associated with an absence of development of pulmonary vascularisation and the parenchyma that depends on it. Secondly, the pulmonary vasculature in the embryo is initially of the systemic type, then progressively the systemic vessels regress and the pulmonary vasculature develops. Consequently, arrest of development of a pulmonary artery or vein responsible for pulmonary hypoplasia does not result in arrest of bronchial development, but in a defect in lung development with persistence of systemic vascularisation. Lobar agenesis and aplasia are the equivalent of lobectomy during foetal life.

In lobar agenesis, the lobar bronchus is completely absent; in lobar aplasia, there is a blind bronchial cul de sac. Pulmonary hypoplasia is characterised by a reduction in the number of bronchial divisions and a defect in the development of the pulmonary parenchyma with a reduction in the number of alveoli. Pulmonary hypoplasia may be primary or secondary to an associated pathology.

Secondary pulmonary hypoplasias are the most common, and many causes have been described, including diaphragmatic hernias, thoracic bone dystrophies, congenital heart disease and renal malformations. Primary pulmonary hypoplasia is due to a defect in the development of the pulmonary vessels: absence of a right or left pulmonary artery or, more exceptionally, right or left pulmonary veins.

XI.1 Lobar **agenesis or aplasia**

They are more frequent on the right than on the left, and the upper lobe is most often affected. They are frequently associated with abnormal pulmonary venous return. Various partial anomalous pulmonary venous returns have been described, the most classic form being Scimitar syndrome or venolobar syndrome in which there is abnormal venous drainage from the right lung into the inferior vena cava. The left-right shunt produced by the venous anomaly is variable and may lead to clinical signs, especially if there is an associated cardiac malformation. Other malformations have been reported: skeletal malformations, bronchopulmonary malformations, retrotracheal left pulmonary artery, accessory diaphragm, sequestration with abnormal pulmonary venous return resulting in Halasz syndrome.

Imaging :

The antenatal diagnosis of these malformations has not been described. Postnatally, the frontal chest X-ray shows a small lung. The reduction in lung volume results in a shift of the mediastinum towards the pathological side, with an elevation of the diaphragmatic dome and relative pinching of the intercostal spaces.

We describe this small lung as "disharmonious". The "disharmonious" character is linked to a partial effacement of the edge of the heart, sometimes associated with an elevation of the diaphragmatic dome, a dense retrosternal band and a venous return anomaly. On the left, the disharmonious character may be due to the presence of an apical cap. The profile X-ray shows the dense retrosternal band. This dense band is created by the line of tangency between the anterior edge of the lung and the deviated mediastinum. This dense band is not always present but is characteristic of lobar agenesis or aplasia. Abnormalities of venous return appear as a vertical, linear or serpentine opacity behind or in contact with the edge of the heart on the frontal X-ray.

Computed tomography with multiplanar and three-dimensional reconstructions confirms the diagnosis by showing the absence of an upper lobar bronchus. It is used to differentiate between agenesis and aplasia when there is a blind cul de sac, and to look for pulmonary venous return anomalies and other bronchopulmonary malformations. Angiography is only performed in cases of associated cardiac disease or in the presence of clinical signs. In practice, the only differential diagnosis is atelectasis.

XI.2 Pulmonary hypoplasia due to defective development of the pulmonary vasculature.

These malformations may be associated with heart disease.

The X-ray shows a small lung which we describe as a "harmonious" small lung, meaning that the edges of the heart are clear, the diaphragmatic dome is normal and there is no dense retrosternal band on the profile.

Unilateral absence of the pulmonary artery is always proximal, due to either agenesis or localised atresia. The anomaly is more common on the left side.

Clinical :

Unilateral absence of the pulmonary artery may be asymptomatic or revealed by signs of pulmonary hypertension or, more rarely, haemoptysis. One complication is worth noting: mountain pulmonary oedema. At mid-altitude, these children may develop pulmonary oedema, which rapidly subsides on their return to the plains. These children are therefore advised to live on the plains.

Imaging :

X-rays show a small, harmonious lung, often hyperclear but without expiratory trapping. The pulmonary hilum is small and there are reticular opacities associated with persistent systemic vascularisation. In older children, costal notches may be seen due to the development of collateral systemic circulation. The aortic arch is located on the right if there is no left pulmonary artery. Lung scans show an absence of perfusion and normal ventilation on the pathological side. A CT scan or MRI can confirm the diagnosis by showing the absence of a pulmonary artery. Unilateral absence of pulmonary veins is exceptional. X-rays show a small harmonious lung, the presence of reticular opacities related to the persistence of systemic vascularisation, and filling of the costo-diaphragmatic cul-de-sac due to the development of sub pleural collateral venous circulation. As with unilateral absence of pulmonary arteries, lung scans show an absence of perfusion and normal ventilation on the pathological side. A CT or MRI scan can confirm the diagnosis by showing the absence of a pulmonary vein. The homolateral pulmonary artery is small and circulates retrogradely.

XII.   Tracheal bronchi

Tracheal bronchi are defined as bronchi arising directly from the trachea or from the stem bronchus upstream of the upper lobar bronchus. The right tracheal bronchi are the most common. Two types have been described: sliding tracheal bronchi, which are the most common, and supernumerary tracheal bronchi. In sliding tracheal bronchi, the lobar bronchus has only two divisions. In supernumerary tracheal bronchi, the lobar bronchus has one normal division.

Clinically, tracheal bronchi are usually asymptomatic and are discovered by chance.

However, they may be associated with chronic cough or recurrent lung infections. The right tracheal bronchus may be revealed by segmental pulmonary condensation of the right upper lobe.

However, the most frequent mode of revelation is an accidental discovery on CT scan.

In exceptional cases, the left tracheal bronchus may develop obstructive emphysema in the area it ventilates, usually the apico-dorsal area. The emphysema is secondary to proximal stenosis of the left tracheal bronchus in contact with the left pulmonary artery.

References

1. k.Bousetta, N.Aloui-kasbi, Z.fitouri. malformations pulmonaires congénitales.Apport de l'imagerie. 17th ed. 27 Apr 2004;

2   Masson E. Physiology of the fetus and newborn - adaptation to extrauterine life [Internet]. EM-Consulte. [cited 23 Oct 2022]. Available from: https://www.em-consulte.com/article/1173319/physiologie-du-fŒtus-et-du-nouveau-ne-adaptation-a

3   Masson E. Embryology [Internet]. EM-Consulte. [cited 23 Oct 2022]. Available from: https://www.em-consulte.com/article/252196/embryologie

4   Masson E. Bronchopulmonary malformations [Internet]. EM-Consulte. [cited 23 Oct 2022]. Available from: https://www.em-consulte.com/article/64845/malformations-bronchopulmonaires

5.   Abdallah RB, Bouthour H, Hellal Y, Malek MRB, Gharbi Y, Kaabar N. Les Malformations Broncho-Pulmonaires : Aspects diagnostiques radiologiques et thérapeutiques. Tunis Med. 2013;91:4.

6   Clements BS, Warner JO. Pulmonary sequestration and related congenital bronchopulmonary-vascular malformations: nomenclature and classification based on anatomical and embryological considerations. Thorax. June 1987;42(6):401-8.

7   Achiron R, Hegesh J, Yagel S. Fetal lung lesions: a spectrum of disease. New classification based on pathogenesis, two-dimensional and color Doppler ultrasound: Editorial. Ultrasound Obstet Gynecol. August 2004;24(2):107-14.

8   Cass DL, Quinn TM, Yang EY, Liechty KW, Crombleholme TM, Flake AW, et al. Increased cell proliferation and decreased apoptosis characterize congenital cystic adenomatoid malformation of the lung. J Pediatr Surg. July 1, 1998;33(7):1043-7.

9.   Langston C. New concepts in the pathology of congenital lung malformations. Semin Pediatr Surg. 1 Feb 2003;12(1):17-37.

10.   Lezmi G, Hadchouel A, Khen-Dunlop N, Vibhushan S, Benachi A, Delacourt C. Cystic adenomatoid malformations of the lung: diagnosis, management, pathophysiological hypotheses. Rev Pneumol Clin. 1 August 2013;69(4):190-7.

11.   Morotti RA, Gutierrez MC, Askin F, Profitt SA, Wert SE, Whitsett JA, et al. Expression of thyroid transcription factor-1 in congenital cystic adenomatoid malformation of the lung. Pediatr Dev Pathol Off J Soc Pediatr Pathol Paediatr Pathol Soc. 2000;3(5):455-61.

12.   Volpe MV, Pham L, Lessin M, Ralston SJ, Bhan I, Cutz E, et al. Expression of Hoxb-5 during human lung development and in congenital lung malformations. Birt Defects Res A Clin Mol Teratol. August 2003;67(8):550-6.

13   Morrisey EE, Hogan BLM. Preparing for the first breath: genetic and cellular mechanisms in lung development. Dev Cell. 19 Jan 2010;18(1):8-23.

14   Simonet WS, DeRose ML, Bucay N, Nguyen HQ, Wert SE, Zhou L, et al. Pulmonary malformation in transgenic mice expressing human keratinocyte growth factor in the lung. Proc Natl Acad Sci U S A. 19 Dec 1995;92(26):12461-5.

15.   M U, Pm del M, Fg S, S B, D W, V F. Tracheal occlusion increases the rate of epithelial branching of embryonic mouse lung via the FGF10-FGFR2b-Sprouty2 pathway. Mech Dev [Internet]. Apr 2008 [cited 28 Nov 2022];125(3-4). Available from: https://pubmed.ncbi.nlm.nih.gov/18082381/

16.   Hadchouel-Duvergé A, Lezmi G, de Blic J, Delacourt C. [Congenital lung malformations: natural history and pathophysiological mechanisms]. Rev Mal Respir. Apr 2012;29(4):601-11.

17.   Costa Júnior A da S, Perfeito JAJ, Forte V. Surgical treatment of 60 patients with pulmonary malformations: what have we learned? J Bras Pneumol Publicacao Of Soc Bras Pneumol E Tisilogia. sept 2008;34(9):661-6.

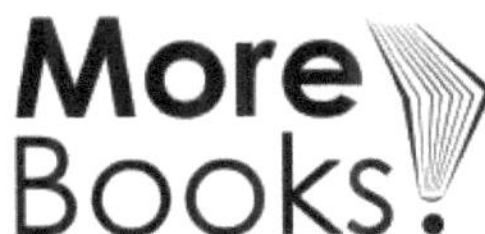

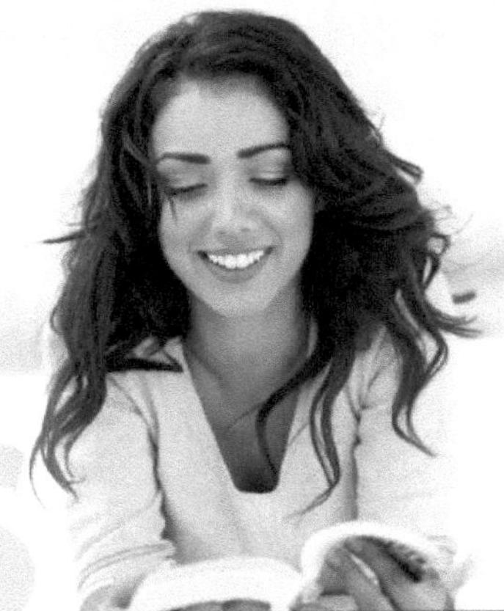

I want morebooks!

Buy your books fast and straightforward online - at one of world's fastest growing online book stores! Environmentally sound due to Print-on-Demand technologies.

Buy your books online at
www.morebooks.shop

Kaufen Sie Ihre Bücher schnell und unkompliziert online – auf einer der am schnellsten wachsenden Buchhandelsplattformen weltweit! Dank Print-On-Demand umwelt- und ressourcenschonend produziert.

Bücher schneller online kaufen
www.morebooks.shop

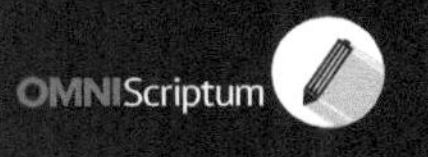

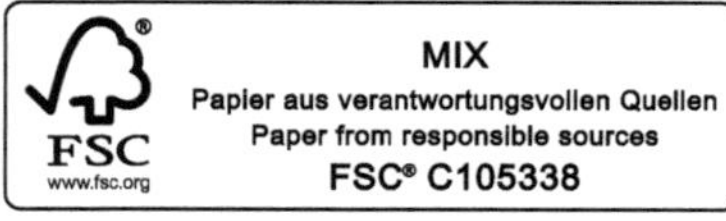

Printed by Books on Demand GmbH, Norderstedt / Germany